YOUR
GUIDE TO ~~~~~~~~~~
GYM WORKOUT

THE DEFINITIVE
GYM COMPANION

By Dr Jonathan S. Lee

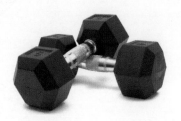

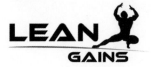

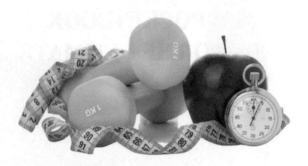

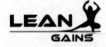

Lean Gains

Copyright © 2020 by Dr. Jonathan S. Lee. All rights reserved.

Book design copyright@2020 ProtectMyWork.com

Visit the author's website at www.leangains.co.uk

Published in United Kingdom

ISBN: 979-857-776-1882 (Paperback)

CONTENTS

ABOUT THE AUTHOR

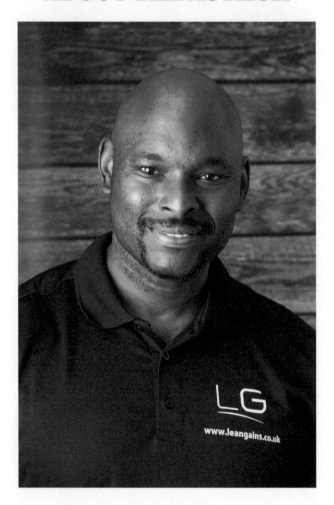

DR JONATHAN S. LEE.....

…is a **qualified sports nutritionist and personal trainer** who has successfully worked with thousands of clients over the past 20 years.

In his early twenties, **Dr Lee was clinically obese** with a body fat percentage of 28. He struggled with obesity for over 3 years trying out a multitude of diets and 'get ripped quick' fitness regimes.

When these fad diets and fitness programmes inevitably failed, Dr Lee made the wise decision to study this topic in more detail by going to university. He graduated from **King's College London in 1998 with a Bachelor of Science in Nutrition and Medical Science**.

He spent the next 5 years of his life researching the science behind fat-loss, muscle growth, healthy living, fitness, and weight training.

In the meantime, he was able to burn **18% body fat in only 10 months!!** This incredible achievement was a strong enough incentive to become a personal trainer in 1999 to help other people reach their fitness goals. He wrote his first book 'Lean Gains' in 2016 and has since written **6 more health and fitness books**.

For more information, visit www.leangains.co.uk

ABOUT THIS BOOK

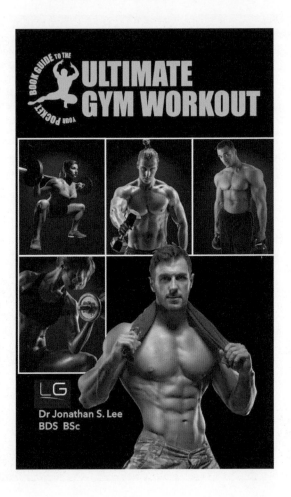

WHAT WILL <u>YOU</u> GET
FROM THIS BOOK?

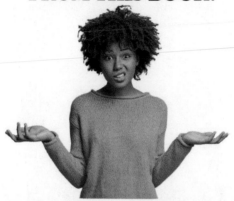

'Your Pocketbook Guide to The Ultimate Gym Workout'
is an adjunct to its parent book **'The Ultimate Gym
Workout.'**

This book sets in place <u>**tried-and-tested**</u>, duplicatable
workouts that are specifically designed to make the most
of your gym sessions and guarantee that you start making
'lean gains.'

This book contains **tailored 3-day and 5-day
workouts** for both men and women, **cardio workouts**,
and stretching routines.

'Your Pocketbook Guide to The Ultimate
Gym Workout' is an absolute <u>**MUST**</u>
for **all** gym enthusiasts.

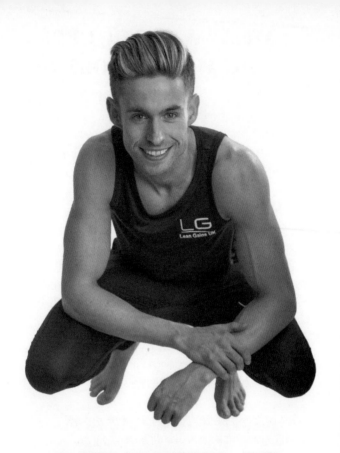

A HANDFUL OF TESTIMONIALS

CHRIS

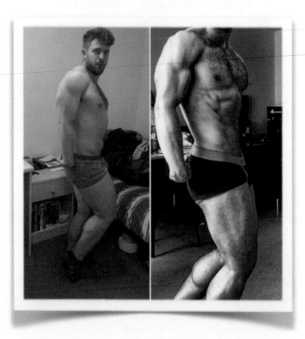

"The training and dieting regimes highlighted throughout this book are essential for success.."

MICHAEL

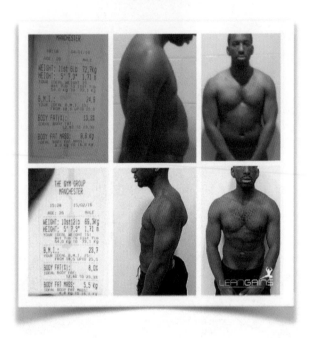

"I lost 8 pounds in 6 weeks and am more than happy with the results. Everything I did to get there is explained in this book!"

JAMIE

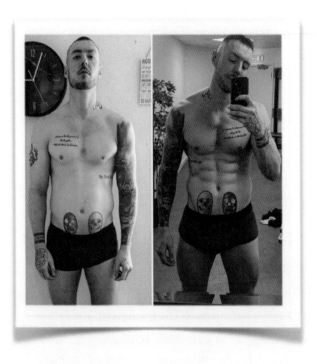

"Speaking as a professional personal trainer, I can say that the advice in Dr Lee's books are spot on!"

SARAH

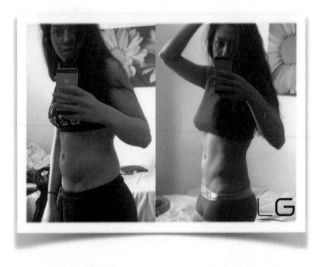

"I am so happy with these results! I've struggled in the past with weight-loss plateaus, but have finally reached may goals!"

SIAN

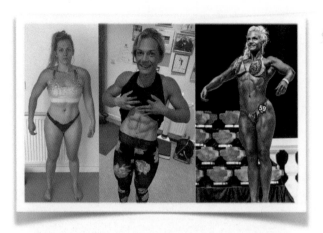

"As a female bodybuilder, I can say that "Your Pocketbook Guide to The Ultimate Gym Workout" is the perfect adjunct for those serious about making some lean gains.!"

MOLLY

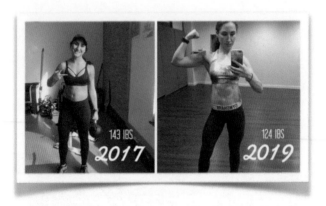

143 IBS
2017

124 IBS
2019

*"'The Ultimate Gym Workout' is an
absolute must for those looking to make
some 'lean gains!'"*

JON

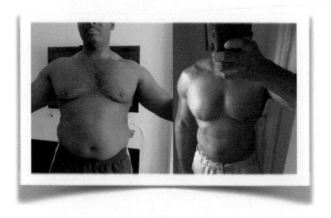

"The routines in this book enabled me to loose 10% body fat in 10 weeks! Strongly recommended"

MICHELLE

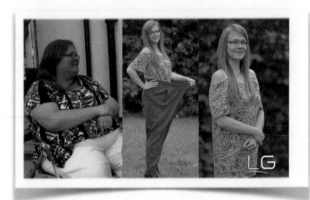

"*I was over 21 stone, and I lost 12 stone in weight in under 2 years. The nutritional advice and dieting regimes in all of Dr. Lee's books are spot on!* "

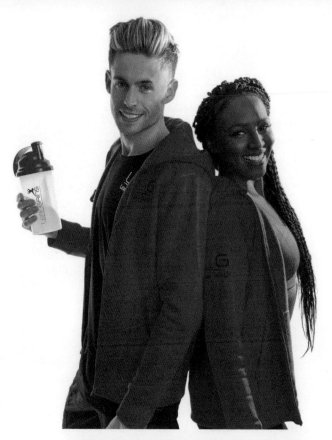

DESIGNING AN
EFFECTIVE
PROGRAMME

1

<u>DESIGNING AN EFFECTIVE PROGRAMME</u>

An effective and sustainable gym routine has to **embrace weight training**, whereby the long-term focus revolves around *progressive overload* and *time-under-tension*.

You should also include some **cardiovascular exercise** (or cardio) into your routine.

It is paramount, however, to undergo a thorough **warm-up** beforehand, irrespective of your workout, in order to get the muscles ready for the gruelling session ahead. Failure to warm up properly can (and often does) lead to injury.

....Oh, and one more thing you can add to the list. A touch of **muscle confusion**. Muscle confusion revolves around the idea of growing muscle by changing your workouts every so often.

The truth is that there's **very little evidence** to suggest that regularly changing your workout regime is any better than applying tried-and-tested methods such as progressive overload to your routine.

However, it does have its place, especially when it comes to directly (or indirectly) working out smaller muscles that are sometimes neglected.

<u>**BABY STEPS ARE EVERYTHING!!!!**</u>

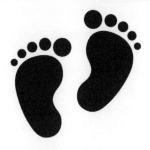

The best way to achieve success in any and every endeavour you do in life is to:

1) Plan what you're doing in advance,

2) Remain focussed and consistent,

3) Gradually progress and improve.

The same is true when it comes to the gym. This is why it's paramount that you apply these principles to your workouts.

The following page shows examples of how you can apply progressive overload and take baby steps to gradually improve your performance in the gym.

WEIGHT TRAINING EXAMPLES

Aim: <u>To Get A Bigger Chest</u>

Week 1: Bench Press, 6 reps, 80kg
Week 3: Bench Press, 8 reps, 80kg
Week 5: Bench Press, 6 reps, 84kg
Week 8: Bench Press, 8 reps, 84kg
Week 10: Bench Press, 6 reps, 86kg

Aim: <u>To Get Bigger Legs</u>

Week 1: Squats, 6 reps, 80kg
Week 3: Squats, 8 reps, 80kg
Week 5: Squats, 6 reps, 84kg
Week 8: Squats, 8 reps, 84kg
Week 10: Squats, 6 reps, 86kg

The Bottom Line

The actual numbers used in the above examples are arbitrary. The point is to slowly increase the number of reps and weight over time. By doing this, your muscles will slowly grow bigger.

CARDIO EXAMPLES

Aim: <u>To Burn Off More Calories</u>

Week 1: Walking, 10 minutes, 2 days/week
Week 2: Walking, 15 minutes 2 days/week
Week 3: Walking, 20 minutes 2 days/week
Week 8: Jogging, 10 minutes 2 days/week
Week 10: Jogging, 15 minutes 2 days/week

Aim: <u>To Burn Off More Calories</u>

Week 1: Slow Cycling, 10 minutes 2 days/week
Week 2: Slow Cycling, 15 minutes 2 days/week
Week 3: Slow Cycling, 20 minutes 3 days/week
Week 6: Faster Cycling, 10 minutes 2 days/week
Week 8: Faster Cycling, 15 minutes 2 days/week
Week 10: Fast Cycling, 15 minutes 2 days/week

The Bottom Line

The actual numbers used in the above examples are arbitrary. The point is to slowly increase the duration and/or intensity on a gradual basis over time.

DIET: BURNING FAT

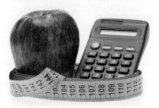

Aim: <u>Burn The Fat, Keep The Muscle</u>

1. Calculate Maintenance Calories
2. Reduce Calorie Intake by 15%
3. Consume Enough Protein = 1g/pound
4. Consume Enough Fat = 0.3-0.5g/pound
5. Consume Enough Fibre = 30g/day
6. Remaining Calories Come From Carbohydrates.

The 'Lean Gains' Book Collection

The aim of this book is to focus on **workout regimes, exercise and fitness**. Diet and nutrition is covered in <u>immense</u> detail in my other books. To learn more about your new diet regime, then check out my other books, **'Lean Gains (2nd Edition)**, **'The Essential Guide to Sports Nutrition and Bodybuilding,'** or **'How to Get The Perfect Body.'**

DIET: BUILDING MUSCLE

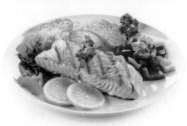

Aim: <u>Build New Muscle with Minimal Fat Gain</u>

1. Calculate Maintenance Calories
2. Increase Calorie Intake by 10%
3. Consume Enough Protein = 1g/pound
4. Consume Enough Fat = 0.3-0.5g/pound
5. Consume Enough Fibre = 30g/day
6. Remaining Calories Come From
   Carbohydrates.

The 'Lean Gains' Book Collection

The aim of this book is to focus on **workout regimes, exercise and fitness**. Diet and nutrition is covered in <u>immense</u> detail in my other books. To learn more about your new diet regime, then check out my other books, **'Lean Gains (2nd Edition), 'The Essential Guide to Sports Nutrition and Bodybuilding,'** or **'How to Get The Perfect Body.'**

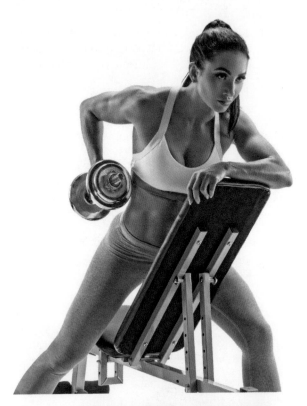

YOUR <u>NEW</u> WORKOUT REGIME

__THE MUSCLES WE NEED__
__TO FOCUS ON__

- Your NEW workout regime will consist of **weight training** and **cardiovascular exercise (cardio)**.

- When it comes to weight training, your workouts will revolve around 8 different parts of the body:

CHEST	**BICEPS**
SHOULDERS	**TRICEPS**
LEGS & CALVES	**ABS**
BACK	**BUTT**

- There are many popular exercises out there that target muscles in these areas. However, quality is more important than quantity.

- The great thing about the workouts in this book is that they're simple yet highly effective. It really is not my aim to bombard you with a ton of exercises that won't necessarily benefit your long-term goals.

HOW WILL THIS NEW WORKOUT REGIME BENEFIT YOU?

THE METHOD BEHIND THE MADNESS

If you go back to page 2, you'll be reminded of all the requirements necessary for an effective programme.

My aim here was to construct a tried-and-tested workout regime that not only ticks all the boxes, but is also simple, duplicatable, and, above all, works to a tee.

Before   After

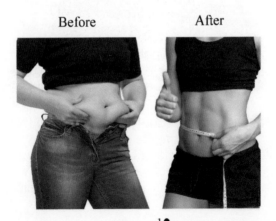

<u>WEIGHT TRAINING</u>

- Our principle goal is to grow and preserve muscle. This is best achieved by firstly **warming up** for 5 to 10 minutes. Doing this reduces risk of injury. You can then start off your main workout with the **heavy duty workouts**, usually comprising of compound exercises using relatively heavy weights.

<u>The Essentials</u>

- Once you've **warmed up**, always start your workout with the **'essential exercises.'**

- The focus of the 'essential' exercises is **progressive overload**.

- Do **ALL** of the 'essential' exercises in the order that they're written.

- Remember, the focus of the 'essential' exercises is progressive overload, so try to **add slightly more weight** each week, if possible, until you're struggling to reach the maximum rep range for that exercise. If you can't add more weight, then focus on doing **more reps** with the same weight.

The Extras

·**Once you've done the essential exercises**, you can then choose 2 to 4 exercises of your choice from the 'extras.'

· The focus of the '**extra**' exercises is **time-under-tension and some muscle confusion**.

· You can get away with just focusing on the essentials to some degree, but the **'extra'** exercises will challenge the muscles in a different way.

· **Unlike** with the essentials, you can pick and choose up to 4 exercises to perform. Try to change these exercises every week.

· The higher rep ranges mean you can and should use lighter weights here allowing for better control of the weight. This is beneficial when you're trying to prolong the rep by focussing on time under tension.

· The choice of exercises available to you here adds diversity as well as an element of muscle confusion to the session.

<u>CARDIOVASCULAR EXERCISE</u>
<u>(Cardio)</u>

<u>IS CARDIO GOOD OR BAD?</u>

Cardio is an excellent adjunct to your weight training sessions, especially if you're looking at burning off any unsightly fat.

Cardio also helps keep you fit and supple. However, doing **too much cardio**, in addition to the intense workout regimes suggested in this book, may contribute towards overtraining.

Therefore, in order to avoid overtraining, it's best to limit your cardio sessions to **no more than 3 x 45 minute cardio sessions a week on top of the workouts suggested**. This is especially the case when it comes to high intensity cardio such as sprinting, insanity-style workouts.

Also, try to do your cardio sessions at least 6 hours before or ideally after your weight training sessions to, again, avoid overtraining/burning out.

And remember what I said on page 9 about baby steps. That's very important here.

<u>YOUR WORKOUT ROUTINE</u>

In this section, we will give a synopsis of the workout routines you will be doing.

They've been divided into **6 sections**.

1) BEGINNER'S WORKOUT

2) WARM UPS

3) OPTION A: THE 5-DAY WORKOUT

4) OPTION B: THE 3-DAY WORKOUT

5) DELOAD WEEK

6) TRACKING YOUR PROGRESS

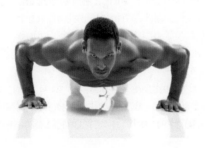

BEGINNER'S WORKOUT

When we bear in mind the relevance of taking baby steps, it is important to keep things simple in the beginning, and progress gradually on a consistent basis.

This is why the **'beginner's workout'** must precede the more challenging workout regimes highlighted in **Options A and B**.

So, Who Is A Beginner?

A beginner is someone who either has never trained with weights before, or very rarely undertakes any weight training.

Even a regular gym-goer can be classed a beginner (or more accurately a 'de-trained weightlifter') if they have been out of the game for a while.

So, Why Are Beginners Treated Differently?

Lifting weights is crucial for maintaining muscle during fat loss and maintenance phases of your diet. Growing muscle when you're on a calorie-surplus also requires a rigorous weight training regime.

The most effective way of benefiting from weight-training in the long-term is by, therefore, setting in place a basis for our training routines.

So, why then are beginners treated differently?

Because:

- These training routines will appear foreign to the **untrained or detrained body**. A beginner should therefore not rush into a conventional strength-training programme. It's better for a beginner to adopt the necessary movements required for muscle growth.

This is why beginners should use relatively light weights for their first month or 2 whilst focussing on compound exercises. Being able to do this serves 2 purposes:

1. It provides the trainee with a foundation from which they can eventually add more weight, build muscle, and become gradually stronger whilst minimising risk of injury.

2. Using light weights from the very beginning allows the trainee to get used to training the right way, optimise their coordination, form a better mind-muscle connection, and hence undergo the required exercises with excellent form.

A workout for a beginner, using this programme, is pretty basic and essentially consists of 2 different workouts on alternate days 3 times a week.

WARMING UP ROUTINES

How Should You Warm Up?

The aim here is to **gradually increase blood flow to the working muscles** by making **incremental** increases in weight from light-to-heavy.

Warming up this way enables your body to perform at a much **greater** intensity when it comes to performing your **working sets**.

Doing a 3-5-minute light jog on a treadmill increases blood flow around the body which better prepares you for the potentially intense upcoming workout.

Once you decide which exercise you're going to do, you can follow up from this 5 minute jog with 10-12 reps at 50% of the weight you would usually lift for a set of 4-6 reps.

This works out at an RPE of around 5.

You can then repeat this and then gradually increase the intensity for another set or 2 before diving into the working sets. You don't need to do more than 4 warm up sets. Remember, you need **enough energy** to perform the working sets!!!

So let's say you've just entered the gym and want to do bench press. Start off with a light jog or cycle at a gentle pace for 5 minutes. Then, if you usually lift 120kg for a set of 4-6 reps, then start off with around 60kg for10-12 reps. **This works out to be 50% intensity of your working set.**

The bottom line is that you should be lifting a weight that's very easy to move about.

Have a break for around a minute and then repeat. By this stage, you should go from **feeling cold and stiff to feeling loose and energised**.

Important Tips About Warming Up?

- **Always** do a warm-up before training each muscle group. For instance, if you're doing legs and back in one session, do a warm up for legs and then do a warm up for back once you've finished training legs.

- **Warm-up on the first exercise you're doing for each muscle group**. So if your first exercise, for instance, is military press, then warm-up on the military press [which trains your shoulders]. If you choose to move onto the next shoulder exercises, once you've completed the military press, you don't need to warm-up again. However, if you decide to train your back afterwards by doing deadlifts, for example, then warm-up on the deadlifts.

- The '**beginner's warm-up regime**' varies slightly to the other warm ups highlighted within this book.

<u>OPTION A: 5-DAY WORKOUT</u>

This workout routine comprises of **five days in the gym and two days of rest**. During each workout routine, emphasis will be placed on two major muscle groups.

<u>OPTION B: 3-DAY WORKOUT</u>

This workout routine comprises of **three days in the gym and four days of rest**. Option B is more suited for those who prefer **not** to train five days a week. The emphasis is placed on three muscle groups per session.

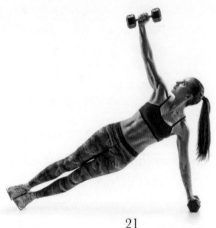

<u>YOUR OCCASIONAL</u>
<u>'DELOAD' WEEK</u>

This **'deload' week** consists of doing **'beginner-style' workouts** consisting of 10-12 reps for 1 week. These exercises are <u>intentionally</u> designed to consist of **relatively simple** and **light** workouts inflicting minimal stress to the muscles.

Lifting 'heavy' all the time creates **immense physical stress** on the body after a while, so it's essential to include a 'de-load' at the end of each training cycle [i.e., **every two months or so**] and let the body rest from strength-training for a while.

That way, when you're ready to go heavy again, the muscles have been well-rested and are rearing to go.

When embarking on a de-load week, ensure that you're using **relatively light weights** throughout.

The alternative to a de-load is to refrain from any weight-training at all for a week and just rest completely.

TRACKING YOUR PROGRESS

Once you get into the habits of performing the workouts in this book, your muscles will naturally become bigger and stronger over time.

Since muscle growth is a gradual progress, any gains in strength and size may not be visually apparent unless you take photos of yourself on a regular basis and document them.

The other obvious method of tracking your progress is by <u>recording and documenting your lifts</u>.

The weights you should make a note of are the ones exclusive to the working sets for the <u>essential</u> workouts only.

The following workouts include tables which allow you to track your progress on a weekly basis.

Alternatively, feel free to download the **'Track Your Progress in The Gym'** pdf from **www.leangains.co.uk**

A FEW MORE WORDS
BEFORE WE GET STUCK IN

- The exercises and routines covered in this book are not an exhaustive list. You may come across '**new**' exercises that aren't covered here, and find them beneficial. Feel free **incorporating** a few new exercises into your regime if you so wish. However, this **does not mean** you should detract or ignore the routines outlined in this book.

- These routines are extremely effective and, in conjunction with a good dieting regime, will enable you to achieve fantastic results. By doing these exercises on a regular basis, you will master them.

- However, **this book is intended to be a short**, concise book that can fit into your back pocket acting as a terrific aid to your workouts whilst you're in the gym.

- I **strongly suggest**, therefore, referring to the **parent book** '**The Ultimate Gym Workout**' (available from www.leangains.co.uk) to learn more about the **ins and outs** of how to properly perform the suggested routines within this book.

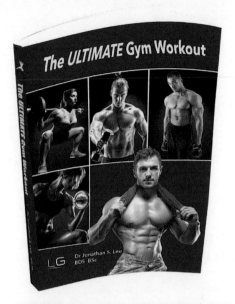

"THE ULTIMATE GYM WORKOUT"

This book sets in place a series of **tried-and-tested** gym workouts whereby all of the exercises are fully explained and illustrated. This eliminates any doubt, with regards to how to perform them, as well as minimising risk of injury associated with poor form and technique.

Available from
www.leangains.co.uk

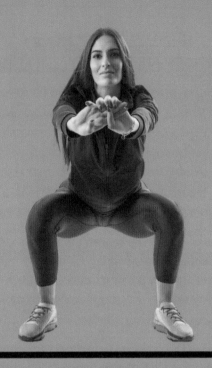

THE
BEGINNER'S
WORKOUT

THE BEGINNER'S WORKOUT

DAY	MAIN FOCUS
MONDAY	CHEST, LEGS, BACK
WEDNESDAY	BACK & SHOULDERS
FRIDAY	CHEST, LEGS, BACK

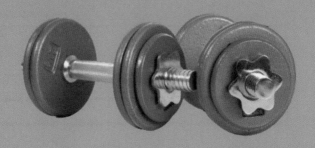

BEGINNER'S

<u>WARM UP</u>

WARMUP SEQUENCE	REP RANGE	INTENSITY (%)	REST
LIGHT CARDIO	3-5 MINUTES	30	
1ST WARMUP SET	10-12 REPS	50	1 minute
2ND WARMUP SET	10-12 REPS	50	1 minute
3RD WARMUP SET	4-6 REPS	70	1 minute
4TH WARMUP SET	1-2 REPS	90-95	3 minutes

MONDAY
BEGINNER'S
WORKOUT

EXERCISE	SETS	REPS	REST
BENCH PRESS	3	8-12	1-2 minutes
SQUATS	3	8-12	1-2 minutes
ROWS	3	8-12	1-2 minutes

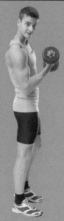
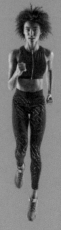

WEDNESDAY
BEGINNER'S
WORKOUT

EXERCISE	SETS	REPS	REST
DEADLIFT	3	8-12	1-2 minutes
LAT PULL DOWNS	3	8-12	1-2 minutes
MILITARY PRESS	3	8-12	1-2 minutes

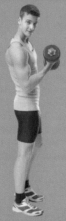
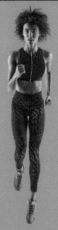

FRIDAY
BEGINNER'S
WORKOUT

EXERCISE	SETS	REPS	REST
BENCH PRESS	3	8-12	1-2 minutes
SQUATS	3	8-12	1-2 minutes
ROWS	3	8-12	1-2 minutes

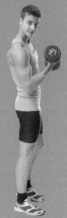
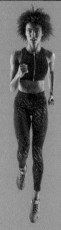

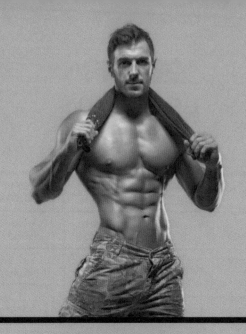

OPTION A

THE 5-DAY
WORKOUT
FOR MEN

THE 5-DAY WORKOUT FOR <u>MEN</u>

DAY	MAIN FOCUS
MONDAY	LEGS & BICEPS
TUESDAY	CHEST & TRICEPS
WEDNESDAY	BACK & ABS
THURSDAY	SHOULDERS & CALVES
FRIDAY	WHOLE BODY
WEEKEND	REST

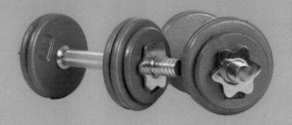

MONDAY

WARM UP

WARMUP SEQUENCE	REP RANGE	INTENSITY (%)	REST
LIGHT CARDIO	3-5 MINUTES	30	
1ST WARMUP SET	10-12 REPS	50	1 minute
2ND WARMUP SET	10-12 REPS	50	1 minute
3RD WARMUP SET	4-6 REPS	70	1 minute
4TH WARMUP SET	1-2 REPS	90-95	3 minutes

MONDAY

<u>THE ESSENTIALS</u>

EXERCISE	SETS	REPS	REST
BARBELL SQUATS	3	4-6	3 minutes
FRONT SQUATS	3	4-6	3 minutes
HIP THRUSTS	3	4-8	3 minutes
ROMANIAN DEADLIFTS	3	4-6	3 minutes
SEATED/ STANDING CALF RAISES	3	8-10	1-2 minutes
DUMBBELL BICEP CURLS	3	4-6	3 minutes
BARBELL CURL	3	6-8	3 minutes

MONDAY

EXTRAS

**PICK 2-4 EXERCISES ONCE
YOU'VE DONE THE ESSENTIALS**

EXERCISE	SETS	REPS	REST
LEG CURL	3	8-12	1-2 minutes
LEG PRESS	3	8-12	1-2 minutes
DUMBBELL/ BARBELL LUNGE	3	8-12	1-2 minutes
HAMMER CURLS	3	8-12	1-2 minutes
CHIN UPS	3	TO FAILURE	1-2 minutes
CALF RAISES ON LEG PRESS	3	8-12	1-2 minutes

MONDAY

TRACK YOUR PROGRESS

USE THE BOXES BELOW TO TRACK YOUR PROGRESS FOR THE 'ESSENTIAL' EXERCISES

EXERCISE	BARBELL SQUATS	FRONT SQUATS	ROMAN. DEADLIFT	CALF RAISE	BICEP CURLS	E-Z BARBELL
WEEK 1						
WEEK 2						
WEEK 3						
WEEK 4						
WEEK5						
WEEK 6						
WEEK 7						
WEEK 8						
WEEK9						
WEEK10						
WEEK 11						
WEEK12						
WEEK 13						
WEEK 14						

TUESDAY

<u>WARM UP</u>

WARMUP SEQUENCE	REP RANGE	INTENSITY (%)	REST
LIGHT CARDIO	3-5 MINUTES	30	
1ST WARMUP SET	10-12 REPS	50	1 minute
2ND WARMUP SET	10-12 REPS	50	1 minute
3RD WARMUP SET	4-6 REPS	70	1 minute
4TH WARMUP SET	1-2 REPS	90-95	3 minutes

TUESDAY

<u>THE ESSENTIALS</u>

EXERCISE	SETS	REPS	REST
FLAT BARBELL BENCHPRESS	3	4-6	3 minutes
INCLINED DUMBBELL/ BARBELL BENCH PRESS	3	4-6	3 minutes
CLOSE-GRIP BENCH PRESS	3	4-6	3 minutes
SKULL CRUSHER	3	6-8	3 minutes
FACEPULL	3	8-12	1-2 minutes

TUESDAY
EXTRAS

**PICK 2-4 EXERCISES ONCE
YOU'VE DONE THE ESSENTIALS**

EXERCISE	SETS	REPS	REST
DIPS	3	8-10	1-2 minutes
DUMBBELL FLYES	3	8-10	1-2 minutes
DUMBBELL PULLOVER	3	8-10	1-2 minutes
TRICEP PRESS	3	8-12	1-2 minutes
TRICEPS PUSHDOWN	3	12-15	1-2 minutes
CABLE CROSSOVER	3	10-12	1-2 minutes
DUMBBELL FLYES	3	10-12	1-2 minutes
INTERNAL/ EXTERNAL DUMBBELL ROTATION	3	8-12	1-2 minutes

TUESDAY

TRACK YOUR PROGRESS

USE THE BOXES BELOW TO TRACK YOUR PROGRESS FOR THE 'ESSENTIAL' EXERCISES

EXERCISE	FLAT BARBELL BENCH PRESS	INCLINED DUMBBELL/ BARBELL BENCH PRESS	CLOSE-GRIP BENCH PRESS	SEATED TRICEP PRESS	FACEPULL
WEEK 1					
WEEK 2					
WEEK 3					
WEEK 4					
WEEK5					
WEEK 6					
WEEK 7					
WEEK 8					
WEEK9					
WEEK10					
WEEK 11					
WEEK12					
WEEK 13					
WEEK 14					

41

WEDNESDAY

WARM UP

WARMUP SEQUENCE	REP RANGE	INTENSITY (%)	REST
LIGHT CARDIO	3-5 MINUTES	30	
1ST WARMUP SET	10-12 REPS	50	1 minute
2ND WARMUP SET	10-12 REPS	50	1 minute
3RD WARMUP SET	4-6 REPS	70	1 minute
4TH WARMUP SET	1-2 REPS	90-95	3 minutes

WEDNESDAY

THE ESSENTIALS

EXERCISE	SETS	REPS	REST
BARBELL DEADLIFT	3	4-6	3 minutes
BARBELL ROW	3	4-6	3 minutes
WIDE-GRIP PULL UP	3	4-6	3 minutes
CABLE CRUNCH	3	4-6	1 minute
HANGING LEG RAISES	3	TO FAILURE	1 minute
AIR BIKE	3	TO FAILURE	1 minute
AB ROLLERS	3	TO FAILUE	1 minute

WEDNESDAY

<u>EXTRAS</u>

**PICK 2-4 EXERCISES ONCE
YOU'VE DONE THE ESSENTIALS**

EXERCISE	SETS	REPS	REST
ONE-ARM DUMBBELL ROW	3	8-10	1-2 minutes
BARBELL/ DUMBBELL SHRUG	3	8-12	3 minutes
LAT PULLDOWN	3	8-12	1-2 minutes
T-BAR ROW	3	8-12	1-2 minutes
HYPER-EXTENSION	3	8-12	1-2 minutes
LEG RAISES	3	TO FAILURE	1-2 minutes

WEDNESDAY

TRACK YOUR PROGRESS

USE THE BOXES BELOW TO TRACK YOUR PROGRESS FOR THE 'ESSENTIAL' EXERCISES

EXERCISE	BARBELL DEADLIFT	BARBELL ROW	WIDE GRIP PULL UP	CABLE CRUNCH
WEEK 1				
WEEK 2				
WEEK 3				
WEEK 4				
WEEK5				
WEEK 6				
WEEK 7				
WEEK 8				
WEEK9				
WEEK10				
WEEK11				
WEEK12				
WEEK13				
WEEK14				

THURSDAY

WARM UP

WARMUP SEQUENCE	REP RANGE	INTENSITY (%)	REST
LIGHT CARDIO	3-5 MINUTES	30	
1ST WARMUP SET	10-12 REPS	50	1 minute
2ND WARMUP SET	10-12 REPS	50	1 minute
3RD WARMUP SET	4-6 REPS	70	1 minute
4TH WARMUP SET	1-2 REPS	90-95	3 minutes

THURSDAY
THE ESSENTIALS

EXERCISE	SETS	REPS	REST
MILITARY PRESS	3	4-6	3 minutes
SIDE LATERAL RAISE	3	4-6	3 minutes
BARBELL REAR DELT ROW	3	4-6	3 minutes
CALF RAISES (STANDING/ SEATED)	3	4-6	3 minute

THURSDAY

EXTRAS

**PICK 2-4 EXERCISES ONCE
YOU'VE DONE THE ESSENTIALS**

EXERCISE	SETS	REPS	REST
REAR DELT RAISE	3	8-12	1-2 minutes
ARNOLD DUMBBELL PRESS	3	10-15	1-2 minutes
DUMBBELL FRONT RAISE	3	8-12	1-2 minutes
BENT OVER DUMBBELL LATERAL RAISE	3	8-12	1-2 minutes
CALF RAISES ON LEG PRESS MACHINE	3	8-12	1-2 minutes

THURSDAY

TRACK YOUR PROGRESS

USE THE BOXES BELOW TO TRACK YOUR PROGRESS FOR THE 'ESSENTIAL' EXERCISES

EXERCISE	MILITARY PRESS	SIDE LATERAL RAISE	BARBELL REAR DELT ROW	CALF RAISES
WEEK 1				
WEEK 2				
WEEK 3				
WEEK 4				
WEEK5				
WEEK 6				
WEEK 7				
WEEK 8				
WEEK9				
WEEK10				
WEEK11				
WEEK12				
WEEK13				
WEEK14				

FRIDAY

WARM UP

WARMUP SEQUENCE	REP RANGE	INTENSITY (%)	REST
LIGHT CARDIO	3-5 MINUTES	30	

The 'Friday' Workout

It's ideal to train the same muscle groups at least twice per week. This is especially true with the smaller muscles such as the abs, biceps, etc.

However, in order to avoid injury or overtraining, the perspective working muscle should undergo one 'heavy' session (low-rep) and one 'lighter' session (higher rep) to maintain adequate growth.

The 'Friday' workout, in addition to the other routines highlighted above, allows for this to occur. As you can see, the 'Friday' sessions have a higher rep range, and hence relatively lighter weights are indicated here.

FRIDAY
<u>WHOLE BODY</u>

EXERCISE	SETS	REPS	REST
DUMBBELL PULLOVER	3	8-12	2 minutes
LEG PRESS	3	8-12	2 minutes
HAMMER CURL	3	8-12	2 minutes
HYPER EXTENSION	3	8-12	2 minutes
TRICEPS PUSHDOWN	3	8-12	2 minutes
FACEPULL	3	8-12	2 minutes
CAPTAIN CHAIR LEG RAISE	3	8-12	1-2 minutes
AIR BICYCLES	3	TO FAILURE	1 minute
AB ROLLER	3	TO FAILURE	1 minute

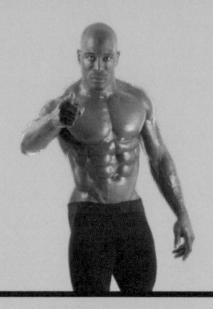

OPTION B

THE 3-DAY
WORKOUT
FOR MEN

THE 3-DAY WORKOUT FOR <u>MEN</u>

DAY	MAIN FOCUS
MONDAY	BACK, ABS & BICEPS
WEDNESDAY	CHEST, TRICEPS & CALVES
FRIDAY	LEGS & SHOULDERS
WEEKEND	REST

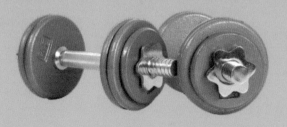

MONDAY

<u>WARM UP</u>

WARMUP SEQUENCE	REP RANGE	INTENSITY (%)	REST
LIGHT CARDIO	3-5 MINUTES	30	
1ST WARMUP SET	10-12 REPS	50	1 minute
2ND WARMUP SET	10-12 REPS	50	1 minute
3RD WARMUP SET	4-6 REPS	70	1 minute
4TH WARMUP SET	1-2 REPS	90-95	3 minutes

MONDAY
<u>THE ESSENTIALS</u>

EXERCISE	SETS	REPS	REST
DEADLIFTS	3	4-6	3 minutes
BARBELL ROW	3	4-6	3 minutes
PULL UPS	3	4-6	3 minutes
BICEP CURLS	3	8-10	3 minutes
HANGING LEG RAISES [weighted if possible]	3	10-12	1-2 minutes
CABLE CRUNCH	3	10-12	1 minutes
AIR BICYCLES	3	TO FAILURE	1 minute

MONDAY

<u>EXTRAS</u>

**PICK 2-4 EXERCISES ONCE
YOU'VE DONE THE ESSENTIALS**

EXERCISE	SETS	REPS	REST
BARBELLL SHRUG	3	8-12	1-2 minutes
HYPER EXTENSION	3	8-12	1-2 minutes
HAMMER CURLS	3	8-12	1-2 minutes
BENT OVER DUMBBELL LATERAL RAISES	3	8-12	1-2 minutes
LAT PULLDOWN	3	12-15	1-2 minutes

MONDAY

TRACK YOUR PROGRESS

USE THE BOXES BELOW TO TRACK YOUR PROGRESS FOR THE 'ESSENTIAL' EXERCISES

EXERCISE	DEADLIFTS	BARBELL ROW	BICEP CURLS	HANGING LEG RAISES WEIGHTED	CABLE CRUNCH
WEEK 1					
WEEK 2					
WEEK 3					
WEEK 4					
WEEK5					
WEEK 6					
WEEK 7					
WEEK 8					
WEEK9					
WEEK10					
WEEK 11					
WEEK12					
WEEK 13					
WEEK 14					

WEDNESDAY

<u>WARM UP</u>

WARMUP SEQUENCE	REP RANGE	INTENSITY (%)	REST
LIGHT CARDIO	3-5 MINUTES	30	
1ST WARMUP SET	10-12 REPS	50	1 minute
2ND WARMUP SET	10-12 REPS	50	1 minute
3RD WARMUP SET	4-6 REPS	70	1 minute
4TH WARMUP SET	1-2 REPS	90-95	3 minutes

WEDNESDAY

<u>THE ESSENTIALS</u>

EXERCISE	SETS	REPS	REST
BENCH PRESS	3	4-6	3 minutes
INCLINED DUMBBELL PRESS	3	4-6	3 minutes
SKULL CRUSHERS	3	4-8	3 minutes
CALF RAISES (Standing/ Seated)	3	4-6	3 minutes

WEDNESDAY
EXTRAS

**PICK 2-4 EXERCISES ONCE
YOU'VE DONE THE ESSENTIALS**

EXERCISE	SETS	REPS	REST
DUMBBELL PULLOVER	3	8-12	1-2 minutes
DIPS	3	8-12	1-2 minutes
CABLE CROSSOVER	3	10-15	1-2 minutes
TRICEPS PUSHDOWN	3	8-12	1-2 minutes
CLOSE-GRIP BENCH PRESS	3	10-15	1-2 minutes
CALF RAISES ON LEG PRESS	3	10-15	1-2 minutes

WEDNESDAY

TRACK YOUR PROGRESS

USE THE BOXES BELOW TO TRACK YOUR PROGRESS FOR THE 'ESSENTIAL' EXERCISES

EXERCISE	BENCH PRESS	INCLINED DUMBBELL	SEATED TRICEP PRESS	CALF RAISES
WEEK 1				
WEEK 2				
WEEK 3				
WEEK 4				
WEEK5				
WEEK 6				
WEEK 7				
WEEK 8				
WEEK9				
WEEK10				
WEEK 11				
WEEK12				
WEEK 13				
WEEK 14				

FRIDAY

<u>WARM UP</u>

WARMUP SEQUENCE	REP RANGE	INTENSITY (%)	REST
LIGHT CARDIO	3-5 MINUTES	30	
1ST WARMUP SET	10-12 REPS	50	1 minute
2ND WARMUP SET	10-12 REPS	50	1 minute
3RD WARMUP SET	4-6 REPS	70	1 minute
4TH WARMUP SET	1-2 REPS	90-95	3 minutes

FRIDAY

<u>THE ESSENTIALS</u>

EXERCISE	SETS	REPS	REST
BARBELL SQUATS	3	4-6	3 minutes
FRONT SQUATS	3	4-6	3 minutes
ROMANIAN DEADLIFT	3	4-6	3 minutes
MILITARY PRESS	3	4-6	3 minutes
BARBELL REAR DELT ROW	3	4-6	3 minutes

FRIDAY

<u>EXTRAS</u>

**PICK 2-4 EXERCISES ONCE
YOU'VE DONE THE ESSENTIALS**

EXERCISE	SETS	REPS	REST
LEG PRESS	3	8-12	1-2 minutes
DUMBBELL/ BARBELL LUNGES	3	8-12	1-2 minutes
DUMBBELL FRONT RAISES	3	10-15	1-2 minutes
ARNOLD DUMBBELL PRESS	3	8-12	1-2 minutes
DUMBBELL SIDE LATERAL RAISES	3	10-15	1-2 minutes
REAR DELT RAISE	3	10-15	1-2 minutes

FRIDAY

TRACK YOUR PROGRESS

USE THE BOXES BELOW TO TRACK YOUR PROGRESS FOR THE 'ESSENTIAL' EXERCISES

EXERCISE	BARBELL SQUATS	FRONT SQUATS	ROMANIAN DEADLIFTS	MILITARY PRESS	BARBELL REAR DELT ROW
WEEK 1					
WEEK 2					
WEEK 3					
WEEK 4					
WEEK5					
WEEK 6					
WEEK 7					
WEEK 8					
WEEK9					
WEEK10					
WEEK 11					
WEEK12					
WEEK 13					
WEEK 14					

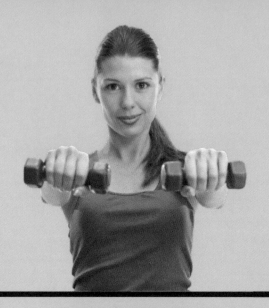

OPTION A

THE 5-DAY WORKOUT FOR WOMEN

THE 5-DAY WORKOUT FOR <u>WOMEN</u>

DAY	MAIN FOCUS
MONDAY	LEGS & BICEPS
TUESDAY	CHEST & TRICEPS
WEDNESDAY	BACK, BUTT & ABS
THURSDAY	SHOULDERS & CALVES
FRIDAY	WHOLE BODY
WEEKEND	REST

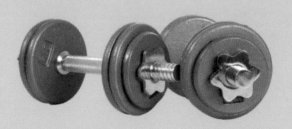

MONDAY

<u>WARM UP</u>

WARMUP SEQUENCE	REP RANGE	INTENSITY (%)	REST
LIGHT CARDIO	3-5 MINUTES	30	
1ST WARMUP SET	10-12 REPS	50	1 minute
2ND WARMUP SET	10-12 REPS	50	1 minute
3RD WARMUP SET	4-6 REPS	70	1 minute
4TH WARMUP SET	1-2 REPS	90-95	3 minutes

MONDAY

THE ESSENTIALS

EXERCISE	SETS	REPS	REST
BARBELL SQUATS	3	4-6	3 minutes
FRONT SQUATS	3	4-6	3 minutes
ROMANIAN DEADLIFTS	3	4-6	3 minutes
HIP THRUSTS	3	4-8	3 minutes
SEATED CALF RAISES	3	8-10	1-2 minutes

MONDAY

EXTRAS

**PICK 2-4 EXERCISES ONCE
YOU'VE DONE THE ESSENTIALS**

EXERCISE	SETS	REPS	REST
LEG CURL	3	8-12	1-2 minutes
LEG PRESS	3	8-12	1-2 minutes
DUMBBELL/ BARBELL LUNGE	3	8-12	1-2 minutes
BUTT BLASTER/ GLUTE MASTER	3	8-12	1-2 minutes
CALF RAISES ON LEG PRESS MACHINE	3	8-12	1-2 minutes

MONDAY

TRACK YOUR PROGRESS

**USE THE BOXES BELOW TO TRACK YOUR
PROGRESS FOR THE 'ESSENTIAL' EXERCISES**

EXERCISE	BARBELL SQUATS	FRONT SQUATS	ROMAN DEADLIFT	HIP THRUSTS	SEATED CALF RAISES
WEEK 1					
WEEK 2					
WEEK 3					
WEEK 4					
WEEK5					
WEEK 6					
WEEK 7					
WEEK 8					
WEEK9					
WEEK10					
WEEK 11					
WEEK12					
WEEK 13					
WEEK 14					

TUESDAY

<u>WARM UP</u>

WARMUP SEQUENCE	REP RANGE	INTENSITY (%)	REST
LIGHT CARDIO	3-5 MINUTES	30	
1ST WARMUP SET	10-12 REPS	50	1 minute
2ND WARMUP SET	10-12 REPS	50	1 minute
3RD WARMUP SET	4-6 REPS	70	1 minute
4TH WARMUP SET	1-2 REPS	90-95	3 minutes

TUESDAY

<u>THE ESSENTIALS</u>

EXERCISE	SETS	REPS	REST
FLAT BARBELL BENCHPRESS	3	4-6	3 minutes
INCLINED DUMBBELL/ BARBELL BENCH PRESS	3	4-6	3 minutes
CLOSE-GRIP BENCH PRESS	3	4-6	3 minutes
SKULL CRUSHER	3	6-8	3 minutes
FACEPULL	3	8-12	1-2 minutes

TUESDAY

<u>EXTRAS</u>

**PICK 2-4 EXERCISES ONCE
YOU'VE DONE THE ESSENTIALS**

EXERCISE	SETS	REPS	REST
DIPS	3	8-10	1-2 minutes
DUMBBELL FLYES	3	8-10	1-2 minutes
DUMBBELL PULLOVER	3	8-10	1-2 minutes
TRICEP PRESS	3	8-12	1-2 minutes
TRICEPS PUSHDOWN	3	12-15	1-2 minutes
CABLE CROSSOVER	3	10-12	1-2 minutes
DUMBBELL FLYES	3	10-12	1-2 minutes
INTERNAL/ EXTERNAL DUMBBELL ROTATION	3	8-12	1-2 minutes

TUESDAY

TRACK YOUR PROGRESS

USE THE BOXES BELOW TO TRACK YOUR PROGRESS FOR THE 'ESSENTIAL' EXERCISES

EXERCISE	FLAT BARBELL BENCH PRESS	INCLINED DUMBBELL/ BARBELL BENCH PRESS	CLOSE-GRIP BENCH PRESS	SEATED TRICEP PRESS	FACEPULL
WEEK 1					
WEEK 2					
WEEK 3					
WEEK 4					
WEEK5					
WEEK 6					
WEEK 7					
WEEK 8					
WEEK9					
WEEK10					
WEEK 11					
WEEK12					
WEEK 13					
WEEK 14					

WEDNESDAY

<u>WARM UP</u>

WARMUP SEQUENCE	REP RANGE	INTENSITY (%)	REST
LIGHT CARDIO	3-5 MINUTES	30	
1ST WARMUP SET	10-12 REPS	50	1 minute
2ND WARMUP SET	10-12 REPS	50	1 minute
3RD WARMUP SET	4-6 REPS	70	1 minute
4TH WARMUP SET	1-2 REPS	90-95	3 minutes

WEDNESDAY

<u>THE ESSENTIALS</u>

EXERCISE	SETS	REPS	REST
BARBELL DEADLIFT	3	4-6	3 minutes
BARBELL ROW	3	4-6	3 minutes
WIDE-GRIP PULL UP	3	4-6	3 minutes
CABLE CRUNCH	3	10-12	1 minute
HANGING LEG RAISES	3	TO FAILURE	1 minute
AIR BIKE	3	TO FAILURE	1 minute
AB ROLLERS	3	TO FAILUE	1 minute

WEDNESDAY

<u>EXTRAS</u>

**PICK 2-4 EXERCISES ONCE
YOU'VE DONE THE ESSENTIALS**

EXERCISE	SETS	REPS	REST
ONE-ARM DUMBBELL ROW	3	8-10	1-2 minutes
BARBELL/ DUMBBELL SHRUG	3	8-12	3 minutes
LAT PULLDOWN	3	8-12	1-2 minutes
T-BAR ROW	3	8-12	1-2 minutes
HYPER-EXTENSION	3	8-12	1-2 minutes
LEG RAISES	3	TO FAILURE	1-2 minutes

WEDNESDAY

TRACK YOUR PROGRESS

USE THE BOXES BELOW TO TRACK YOUR PROGRESS FOR THE 'ESSENTIAL' EXERCISES

EXERCISE	BARBELL DEADLIFT	BARBELL ROW	WIDE GRIP PULL UP	CABLE CRUNCH
WEEK 1				
WEEK 2				
WEEK 3				
WEEK 4				
WEEK5				
WEEK 6				
WEEK 7				
WEEK 8				
WEEK9				
WEEK10				
WEEK11				
WEEK12				
WEEK13				
WEEK14				

THURSDAY

<u>WARM UP</u>

WARMUP SEQUENCE	REP RANGE	INTENSITY (%)	REST
LIGHT CARDIO	3-5 MINUTES	30	
1ST WARMUP SET	10-12 REPS	50	1 minute
2ND WARMUP SET	10-12 REPS	50	1 minute
3RD WARMUP SET	4-6 REPS	70	1 minute
4TH WARMUP SET	1-2 REPS	90-95	3 minutes

THURSDAY

<u>THE ESSENTIALS</u>

EXERCISE	SETS	REPS	REST
MILITARY PRESS	3	4-6	3 minutes
SIDE LATERAL RAISE	3	4-6	3 minutes
BARBELL REAR DELT ROW	3	4-6	3 minutes
CALF RAISES (STANDING/ SEATED)	3	4-6	3 minute

THURSDAY

<u>EXTRAS</u>

**PICK 2-4 EXERCISES ONCE
YOU'VE DONE THE ESSENTIALS**

EXERCISE	SETS	REPS	REST
REAR DELT RAISE	3	8-12	1-2 minutes
ARNOLD DUMBBELL PRESS	3	10-15	1-2 minutes
DUMBBELL FRONT RAISE	3	8-12	1-2 minutes
BENT OVER DUMBBELL LATERAL RAISE	3	8-12	1-2 minutes
CALF RAISES ON LEG PRESS MACHINE	3	12-15	1-2 minutes

THURSDAY

TRACK YOUR PROGRESS

**USE THE BOXES BELOW TO TRACK YOUR
PROGRESS FOR THE 'ESSENTIAL' EXERCISES**

EXERCISE	MILITARY PRESS	SIDE LATERAL RAISE	BARBELL REAR DELT ROW	CALF RAISES
WEEK 1				
WEEK 2				
WEEK 3				
WEEK 4				
WEEK5				
WEEK 6				
WEEK 7				
WEEK 8				
WEEK9				
WEEK10				
WEEK11				
WEEK12				
WEEK13				
WEEK14				

FRIDAY

WARM UP

WARMUP SEQUENCE	REP RANGE	INTENSITY (%)	REST
LIGHT CARDIO	3-5 MINUTES	30	

The 'Friday' Workout

It's ideal to train the same muscle groups at least twice per week. This is especially true with the smaller muscles such as the abs, biceps, etc.

However, in order to avoid injury or overtraining, the perspective working muscle should undergo one 'heavy' session (low-rep) and one 'lighter' session (higher rep) to maintain adequate growth.

The 'Friday' workout, in addition to the other routines highlighted above, allows for this to occur. As you can see, the 'Friday' sessions have a higher rep range, and hence relatively lighter weights are indicated here.

FRIDAY

<u>WHOLE BODY</u>

EXERCISE	SETS	REPS	REST
SQUATS	3	8-12	2 minutes
LEG PRESS	3	8-12	2 minutes
HAMMER CURL	3	8-12	2 minutes
HYPER EXTENSION	3	8-12	2 minutes
TRICEPS PUSHDOWN	3	8-12	2 minutes
FACEPULL	3	8-12	2 minutes
CAPTAIN CHAIR LEG RAISE	3	8-12	1-2 minutes
AIR BICYCLES	3	TO FAILURE	1 minute
AB ROLLER	3	TO FAILURE	1 minute

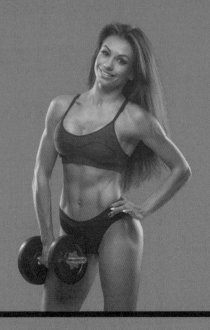

OPTION B

THE 3-DAY
WORKOUT
FOR WOMEN

THE 3-DAY WORKOUT FOR <u>WOMEN</u>

DAY	MAIN FOCUS
MONDAY	BACK, BUTT & ABS
WEDNESDAY	CHEST, TRICEPS & CALVES
FRIDAY	LEGS, BUTT & SHOULDERS
WEEKEND	REST

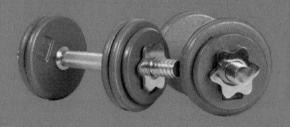

MONDAY

WARM UP

WARMUP SEQUENCE	REP RANGE	INTENSITY (%)	REST
LIGHT CARDIO	3-5 MINUTES	30	
1ST WARMUP SET	10-12 REPS	50	1 minute
2ND WARMUP SET	10-12 REPS	50	1 minute
3RD WARMUP SET	4-6 REPS	70	1 minute
4TH WARMUP SET	1-2 REPS	90-95	3 minutes

MONDAY

<u>THE ESSENTIALS</u>

EXERCISE	SETS	REPS	REST
DEADLIFTS	3	4-6	3 minutes
BARBELL ROW	3	4-6	3 minutes
PULL UPS	3	4-6	3 minutes
BICEP CURLS	3	8-10	3 minutes
BULGARIAN SPLIT SQUATS	3	10-12	1-2 minutes
CABLE CRUNCH	3	10-12	1 minutes
AIR BICYCLES	3	TO FAILURE	1 minute

MONDAY

<u>EXTRAS</u>

**PICK 2-4 EXERCISES ONCE
YOU'VE DONE THE ESSENTIALS**

EXERCISE	SETS	REPS	REST
BARBELLL SHRUG	3	8-12	1-2 minutes
HYPER EXTENSION	3	8-12	1-2 minutes
HAMMER CURLS	3	8-12	1-2 minutes
BENT OVER DUMBBELL LATERAL RAISES	3	8-12	1-2 minutes
LAT PULLDOWN	3	12-15	1-2 minutes

MONDAY

TRACK YOUR PROGRESS

USE THE BOXES BELOW TO TRACK YOUR PROGRESS FOR THE 'ESSENTIAL' EXERCISES

EXERCISE	DEADLIFTS	BARBELL ROW	BICEP CURLS	BULGARIAN SPLIT SQUATS	CABLE CRUNCH
WEEK 1					
WEEK 2					
WEEK 3					
WEEK 4					
WEEK5					
WEEK 6					
WEEK 7					
WEEK 8					
WEEK9					
WEEK10					
WEEK 11					
WEEK12					
WEEK 13					
WEEK 14					

WEDNESDAY

<u>WARM UP</u>

WARMUP SEQUENCE	REP RANGE	INTENSITY (%)	REST
LIGHT CARDIO	3-5 MINUTES	30	
1ST WARMUP SET	10-12 REPS	50	1 minute
2ND WARMUP SET	10-12 REPS	50	1 minute
3RD WARMUP SET	4-6 REPS	70	1 minute
4TH WARMUP SET	1-2 REPS	90-95	3 minutes

WEDNESDAY

THE ESSENTIALS

EXERCISE	SETS	REPS	REST
BENCH PRESS	3	4-6	3 minutes
INCLINED DUMBBELL PRESS	3	4-6	3 minutes
SKULL CRUSHER	3	4-6	3 minutes
CALF RAISES (Standing/ Seated)	3	4-6	3 minutes

WEDNESDAY

EXTRAS

**PICK 2-4 EXERCISES ONCE
YOU'VE DONE THE ESSENTIALS**

EXERCISE	SETS	REPS	REST
DUMBBELL PULLOVER	3	8-12	1-2 minutes
DIPS	3	8-12	1-2 minutes
CABLE CROSSOVER	3	10-15	1-2 minutes
TRICEPS PUSHDOWN	3	8-12	1-2 minutes
CLOSE-GRIP BENCH PRESS	3	10-15	1-2 minutes
CALF RAISES ON LEG PRESS	3	10-15	1-2 minutes

WEDNESDAY

TRACK YOUR PROGRESS

USE THE BOXES BELOW TO TRACK YOUR PROGRESS FOR THE 'ESSENTIAL' EXERCISES

EXERCISE	BENCH PRESS	INCLINED DUMBBELL	SEATED TRICEP PRESS	CALF RAISES
WEEK 1				
WEEK 2				
WEEK 3				
WEEK 4				
WEEK5				
WEEK 6				
WEEK 7				
WEEK 8				
WEEK9				
WEEK10				
WEEK 11				
WEEK12				
WEEK 13				
WEEK 14				

FRIDAY

<u>WARM UP</u>

WARMUP SEQUENCE	REP RANGE	INTENSITY (%)	REST
LIGHT CARDIO	3-5 MINUTES	30	
1ST WARMUP SET	10-12 REPS	50	1 minute
2ND WARMUP SET	10-12 REPS	50	1 minute
3RD WARMUP SET	4-6 REPS	70	1 minute
4TH WARMUP SET	1-2 REPS	90-95	3 minutes

FRIDAY

<u>THE ESSENTIALS</u>

EXERCISE	SETS	REPS	REST
BARBELL SQUATS	3	4-6	3 minutes
FRONT SQUATS	3	4-6	3 minutes
ROMANIAN DEADLIFT	3	4-6	3 minutes
HIP THRUST	3	4-8	3 minutes
MILITARY PRESS	3	4-6	3 minutes

FRIDAY

EXTRAS

**PICK 2-4 EXERCISES ONCE
YOU'VE DONE THE ESSENTIALS**

EXERCISE	SETS	REPS	REST
LEG PRESS	3	8-12	1-2 minutes
DUMBBELL/ BARBELL LUNGES	3	8-12	1-2 minutes
DUMBBELL FRONT RAISES	3	10-15	1-2 minutes
ARNOLD DUMBBELL PRESS	3	8-12	1-2 minutes
DUMBBELL SIDE LATERAL RAISES	3	10-15	1-2 minutes
REAR DELT RAISE	3	10-15	1-2 minutes

FRIDAY

TRACK YOUR PROGRESS

USE THE BOXES BELOW TO TRACK YOUR PROGRESS FOR THE 'ESSENTIAL' EXERCISES

EXERCISE	BARBELL SQUATS	FRONT SQUATS	ROMANIAN DEADLIFTS	HIP THRUST	MILITARY PRESS
WEEK 1					
WEEK 2					
WEEK 3					
WEEK 4					
WEEK5					
WEEK 6					
WEEK 7					
WEEK 8					
WEEK9					
WEEK10					
WEEK 11					
WEEK12					
WEEK 13					
WEEK 14					

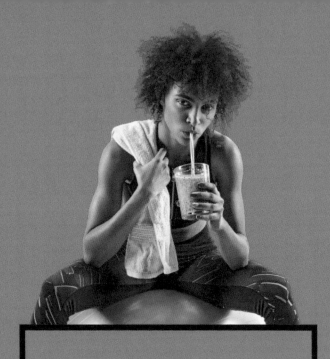

DELOAD
WEEK

DELOAD WEEK

**TO BE DONE APPROXIMATELY
EVERY 8 WEEKS**

DAY	MAIN FOCUS
MONDAY	DELOAD DAY 1
WEDNESDAY	DELOAD DAY 2
FRIDAY	DELOAD DAY 3
WEEKEND	REST

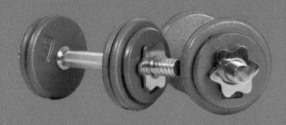

101

DELOAD

<u>WARM UP</u>

WARMUP SEQUENCE	REP RANGE	INTENSITY (%)	REST
LIGHT CARDIO	3-5 MINUTES	30	
1ST WARMUP SET	10-12 REPS	50	1 minute
2ND WARMUP SET	10-12 REPS	50	1 minute
3RD WARMUP SET	4-6 REPS	70	1 minute

MONDAY

<u>DELOAD DAY 1</u>

EXERCISE	SETS	REPS	REST
DEADLIFTS	3	8-12	3 minutes
BARBELL ROW	3	8-12	3 minutes
HANGING LEG RAISES	3	10-12	3 minutes
AB ROLLERS	3	8-10	3 minutes
BULGARIAN SPLIT SQUATS	3	10-12	3 minutes
AIR BICYCLES	3	10-12	2 minutes
AB ROLLERS	3	10-12	2 minute

WEDNESDAY

<u>DELOAD DAY 2</u>

EXERCISE	SETS	REPS	REST
BENCH PRESS	3	8-12	3 minutes
INCLINED DUMBBELL PRESS	3	8-12	3 minutes
MILITARY PRESS	3	10-12	3 minutes

FRIDAY

<u>DELOAD DAY 3</u>

EXERCISE	SETS	REPS	REST
BARBELL SQUATS	3	8-12	3 minutes
FRONT SQUAT	3	8-12	3 minutes
ROMANIAN DEADLIFT	3	8-12	3 minutes
BARBELL CURLS	3	8-12	3 minutes

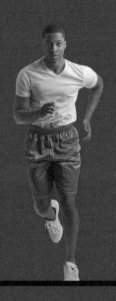

WHAT ABOUT CARDIO?

HOW TO ADD CARDIO TO YOUR WEEKLY ROUTINE

What is Cardio?

Cardiovascular Exercise (or cardio) is any activity that increases heart rate and respiration while using large muscle groups repetitively and rhythmically.

The main reason we do cardio is to help us keep fit and healthy, optimise heart function, and, above all, help us burn more calories (fat).

When it comes to building new muscle and getting ripped, however, cardio is no substitute to the aforementioned training regimes.

There are 3 main types of cardio that you can implement into your regime. They are:

- Low-Intensity Cardio
- High-Intensity Intermittent Training (HIIT)
- Metabolice Resistance Training (MRT)

LOW-INTENSITY CARDIO

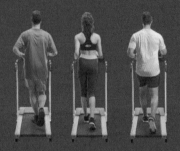

What is Low-Intensity Cardio?

Low-intensity cardio is when you perform low-impact exercises that fulfil all of the cardiovascular benefits of exercise without over-taxing the body.

Examples

Walking, Jogging, Swimming, Rowing, Walking or Light Jogging on a Treadmill, Bike-Riding, etc.

Duration and Frequency

45-60 minutes per session 2 times per week in addition to your weight training regimes should suffice.

HIGH-INTENSITY CARDIO

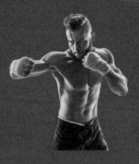

What is HIIT Cardio?

HIIT involves short bursts of intense exercise alternated with low-intensity or recovery periods.

Examples

Boxing, Sprinting, Skipping, Shaun T's Insanity Workout, Circuit Training, etc. HIIT sessions-1 and 2 on the following pages are also great HIIT exercises.

Duration and Frequency

20-30 minutes per session 2-3 times per week in addition to your weight training regimes should suffice.

HIIT SESSION-1

30-SECOND SPRINTS IN A
20 MINUTE HIIT SESSION

EXERCISE	DURATION
WARM-UP (eg. Light jog)	5 minutes
1st SPRINT	30 seconds
Walk/Light Jog	2 minutes
2nd SPRINT	30 seconds
Walk/Light Jog	2 minutes
3rd SPRINT	30 seconds
Walk/Light Jog	2 minutes
4th SPRINT	30 seconds
Walk/Light Jog	2 minutes
5th SPRINT	30 seconds
Walk/Light Jog	2 minutes
6th SPRINT	30 seconds
Cool down/stretch	5 minutes

HIIT SESSION-2

CIRCUIT TRAINING

WHAT IS CIRCUIT TRAINING?

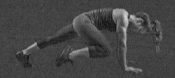

Circuit training is a fast-paced series of exercises whereby you do exercise from around 30-seconds to 2-minutes and then move onto another exercise.

EXERCISE	DURATION
WARM-UP (eg. Light jog)	5 minutes
BURPEES	30 seconds
JUMPING JACKS	30 seconds
SKIPPING	30 seconds
MOUNTAIN CLIMBERS	30 seconds
REST	30 seconds

WHAT ABOUT <u>MRT</u>?

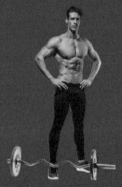

<u>What is MRT?</u>

MRT involves performing resistance and compound exercises at a very rapid pace with little or no rest in between exercises.

<u>What Are The Protocols for MRT?</u>

A Light Weight, Engaging All Muscle Groups (ie. Compound Exercises), and Short Rest Periods (between circuits).

<u>Duration and Frequency</u>

20-30 minutes per session no more than 2 times per week in addition to your weight training regimes should suffice.

A SAMPLE MRT CIRCUIT

HOW TO PERFORM THIS CIRCUIT?

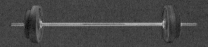

Always start off with a 5-minute light jog. Then using a light-weight (eg. RPE 4), perform the following exercises without rest. Once you've finished the circuit, rest for 2 minutes. Repeat the circuit 5 more times.

EXERCISE	DURATION/REPS
WARM-UP (eg. Light jog)	5 minutes
BENCH PRESS	20 reps
DEADLIFT	20 reps
PULL-UPS	10 reps
OVERHEAD PRESS	20 reps
SQUATS	20 reps
REST	2 minutes

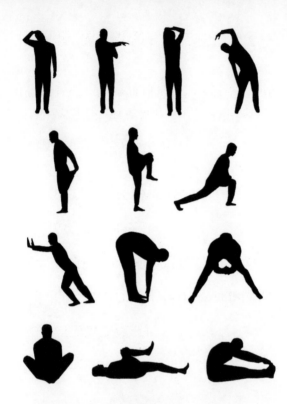

10 ESSENTIAL POST-WORKOUT STRETCHES

HAMSTRINGS

There are many ways by which you can stretch the hamstring muscles and they are all effective. However, my favourite is the 'standing hamstring stretch.'

The Standing Hamstring Stretch

1. Stand up with straight legs, both feet flat on the floor, and knees straight.

2. Lower your forehead towards your knees whilst bending at the waist until you feel the hamstrings stretch.

3. Hold for 20-30 seconds and repeat twice.

    - If you're very flexible, you can rest your hands on the floor.

    - Alternatively, go down as low as you can **without** over-stretching your hamstrings. Aim to touch your toes.

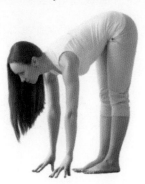

QUADRICEPS

Muscle tension in the **quadriceps** can lead to back and knee pain, overall tightness, and reduced mobility. This is why stretching them is of paramount importance after intense workouts.

Simple Quadricep Stretch

1. Stand upright with feet together.

2. Stand on your left leg whilst grabbing the right leg and pulling it towards your butt. If you're feeling unstable on one leg, you can use a wall or something sturdy to keep yourself steady.

3. Make sure you push your chest up and hips forward whilst holding the position for 20-30 seconds and repeat twice. You should feel a nice stretch in your quads.

4. Repeat using the left leg and right hand.

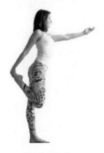

PIRIFORMIS

The piriformis is a small muscle located deep in the buttock, behind the gluteus maximus. The piriformis stretch feels as if you're stretching the gluteal (butt) muscles.

Piriformis and Outer Hip Stretch

1. Lie down on your back, place both feet flat on the floor and bend both knees.

2. Place your left ankle on (or just below) your right knee so that your left ankle is closer to you.

3. Grab your right knee with both hands and pull towards your chest. You will feel a stretch on the left gluteal muscle and back of the left leg when you do this.

4. Hold for 20-30 seconds and repeat twice.

5. Then repeat the above with the right leg.

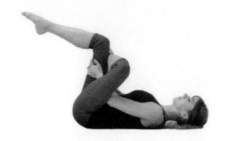

CALF MUSCLES

When the two main calf muscles (the gastrocnemius and the soleus) are tight and inflexible, they might affect your distribution of weight and the pressure you're applying to other areas of your body as you move around.

Simple Calf Stretch

1. Place one foot in front of the other, whilst the front knee is slightly bent. (Alternatively, stand in front of a wall and lean towards it.

2. Keep your back knee and leg straight, your heel on the ground, and lean forwards.

3. Slowly push until you feel a nice stretch inn the calf muscles.

4. Hold for 20-30 seconds, repeat twice and switch legs.

__DELTOIDS__

This exercise helps increase flexibility and range of motion in your shoulder joint and the surrounding muscles. When doing this exercise, lower your arm if you feel any pain in your shoulder.

__Across-The-Chest Stretch__

1. Straighten your right arm and extend your right arm across the chest so the biceps are touching the pecs.

2. Place your left hand onto the crease of the right elbow and pull further towards your chest.

3. Hold this position for 30 seconds.

4. Repeat on the other side.

5. Do each side 3 more times.

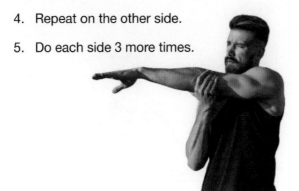

ADDUCTORS

The adductors, often referred to as your groin
muscles, are a group of muscles that sit around
your inner thigh area.

Standing Adductor Stretch

1. Stand with your feet approximately 3 feet apart.

2. Turn towards the right and bend your right knee
   whilst keeping the left leg straight until you feel
   a stretch in the inner part of your left thigh. Try
   to avoid your knee going in front of your toes.

3. Hold for 30 seconds, repeat twice.

4. Repeat the above steps with the left leg bent.

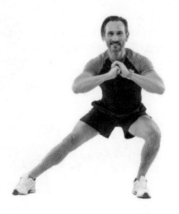

PECTORALIS & BICEPS

This is an excellent stretch following an upper body workout as it will relieve muscle tightness and tension in the biceps, chest and shoulder muscles.

Wall Bicep/Chest Stretch

1. Press your left palm against something sturdy like a wall or post.

2. Ensure your arm is straight and fingers are pointing away from you.

3. Slowly rotate your body away from the wall until you feel a stretch in your chest and biceps.

4. Hold this position for 30 seconds and repeat twice.

5. Switch arms.

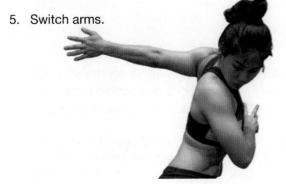

ABDOMINAL

The 'cobra pose' increases the flexibility of the spine. It stretches the chest while strengthening the spine and shoulders. It also helps to open the lungs and stretches the abdominal muscles.

Cobra Pose

1. Lie down on your stomach with your legs straight and **the feet hip-width apart**.

2. Press feet (nails down) into the floor and place palms on the ground next to your rib cage so that **your forearms are vertical.**

3. Inhale as you gently lift your head and chest off the floor. Keep your lower ribs on the floor.

4. Draw your shoulders back, do not crunch your neck. Keep your shoulders dropped away from your ears. Slowly push upwards until you feel an abdominal stretch.

5. Only straighten your arms as much as your body allows. Deepen the stretch as your practice advances, but avoid straining to achieve a deeper backbend.

TRICEPS

The benefits of stretching the triceps are to improve flexibility and increase muscle length, improve function and maintain range of motion around elbows.

Behind-the-Head Triceps Stretch

1. Stand with your back straight and your feet shoulder-width apart. You can do this stretch sitting down if that's more comfortable for you.

2. Lift your right hand straight above your head and bend at the elbow. Keep your chin tucked in.

3. Place your left hand on your right elbow and gently pull down until you feel a stretch in the triceps.

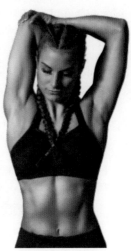

4. Hold in this position for 30 seconds and repeat twice.

5. Switch arms remembering to keep your chin tucked in.

HIPS AND ILITIBIAL (IT) BAND

Your iliotibial band (IT band) is a thickened band of tissue that runs all the way down the length of your thigh. It helps stabilise your knees, but can become very inflamed and tight after prolonged running, cycling or leg exercises.

Seated Hip, Glute and ITB Stretch

1. Sit on the floor with both legs extended in front of you.

2. Cross the right leg over the left so that the right foot is flat on the floor.

3. Place your right hand on the floor behind your body as in the diagram.

4. Place your left hand on your outer right thigh. Alternatively, place your left elbow on the outside of your right knee (if you're flexible enough).

5. Pull your right leg to the left whilst twisting your torso to the right.

6. Hold for 30 seconds and repeat twice. Repeat the above steps using the left leg and the right arm to pull.

124

...IS THAT IT??

- You are probably aware of **other stretches** you can do and add to your routine, and I would strongly encourage you to do so.

- The above 10 stretches, however, will **significantly** reduce the risk of injury in the long term by keeping your muscles and joints flexible and supple.

- Remember to ideally reserve these stretches until after your workout once your muscles are already warm. This reduces the risk of potential injury, and we don't want that.

- However, as with the weight training and cardio sessions, you **must** see a physiotherapist or doctor if you start to feel any discomfort during or after your gym sessions. It's always better to tackle any potential problems early on since the longer you wait, the longer it takes to treat.

- Likewise, **seek medical advice** if you have any pre-existing injuries, heart problems, or any other medical condition, prior to undertaking any of the aforementioned workouts in this book. After all, prevention is always better than cure.

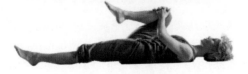

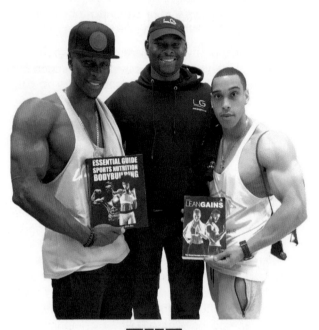

THE
'LEAN GAINS'
BOOK
COLLECTION

<u>WHY NOT CHECK OUT</u>
<u>MY OTHER BOOKS?</u>

Thank you for purchasing:

'Your Pocketbook Guide to The Ultimate Gym Workout.'

If you enjoyed reading this book or would like to purchase another book from the

'Lean Gains Book Collection,'

then please visit my website:

www.leangains.co.uk

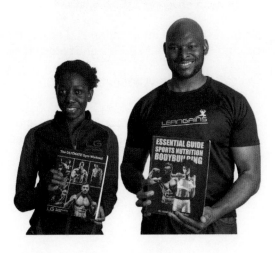

THE ESSENTIAL GUIDE TO SPORTS NUTRITION AND BODYBUILDING

'The Essential Guide to Sports Nutrition and Bodybuilding' contains everything you need to know about losing weight, eating right, gaining muscle, feeling great, and living a long, healthy, and vibrant life.

Outstanding Features include:

- **800 pages** of attractive, easy-to-digest information covering a huge range of topics.

- **Science-backed information** and advice based on over **580 clinical studies and references**.

- Over **254 full-colour photographs** and illustrations.

- Simple descriptions, paragraph breaks, and a **key-point summary** at the end of each chapter to allow for enjoyable reading.

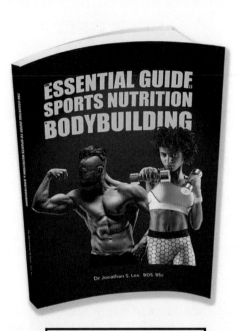

HARDBACK:	£64.99
PAPERBACK:	£49.99
E-BOOK:	£9.99

(prices may vary)

AVAILABLE AT

WWW.LEANGAINS.CO.UK

and

Amazon

LEAN GAINS
(2nd Edition)

'Lean Gains (2nd edition)' is an absolute MUST for those who are struggling to burn fat, bulk up, and break through weight-loss plateaus. Dr Lee has created a comprehensive blueprint to help manage your weight and achieve faster results than you would using conventional dieting methods.

Outstanding Features include:

- **470 pages** of easy-to-digest information relating to the science behind fat-loss and muscle gain.

- **Science-backed information** and advice based on over **500 clinical studies and references**.

- Over **200 full-colour photographs** and illustrations.

- **Paragraph breaks**, colour pictures on almost every page, and a gentle sense of humour for enjoyable reading.

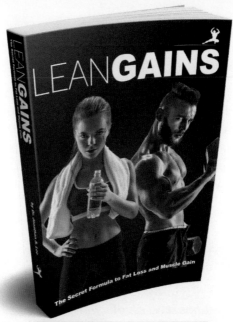

HARDBACK:	£49.99
PAPERBACK:	£45.99
E-BOOK:	£9.99
AUDIOBOOK	£9.99

(prices may vary)

AVAILABLE AT
WWW.LEANGAINS.CO.UK
and
Amazon

THE ULTIMATE GYM WORKOUT

'The Ultimate Gym Workout' is the perfect adjunct to your gym workouts. This book sets in place a series of effective, tried-and-tested gym workouts. Designated set ranges, rep ranges, and rest periods take away the need to focus on anything other than the workouts themselves.

Outstanding Features include:

- **155 full-colour photographs and illustrations.**

- Detailed **weight-training , stretching routines,** and **cardio workouts**.

- Simple descriptions and video links (ebook version).

- **Meal plans** and **nutritional advice**.

- **Exercise routines** tailored for both **men and women**.

- Choice between **3-day and 5-day workouts.**

- All exercise are **fully explained** and **illustrated.**

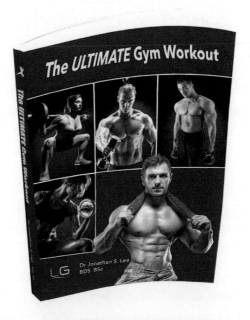

HARDBACK:	N/A
PAPERBACK:	£39.99
E-BOOK:	£9.99

(prices may vary)

AVAILABLE AT
WWW.LEANGAINS.CO.UK
and
Amazon

YOUR POCKETBOOK GUIDE TO THE ULTIMATE GYM WORKOUT

'Your Pocketbook Guide to The Ultimate Gym Workout' is the 'pocketbook' accompaniment to its larger parent book
'The Ultimate Gym Workout.'

This book sets in place a series of effective tried-and-tested gym workouts.

Outstanding Features include:

- Detailed **weight-training, cardio workouts, and stretching routines**.

- Simple descriptions and video links (ebook version).

- **Exercise routines** tailored for both **men and women**.

- Choice between **3-day and 5-day workouts.**

- All exercise are **fully explained** and **illustrated.**

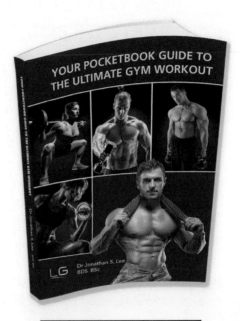

HARDBACK:	N/A
PAPERBACK:	£14.99
E-BOOK:	£9.99

(prices may vary)

AVAILABLE AT
WWW.LEANGAINS.CO.UK
and
Amazon

HOW TO GET THE PERFECT BODY

'How to Get The Perfect Body' is a no-BS introduction to the world of diet and fitness.

'How To Get The Perfect Body'
is extremely easy on the eye, contains a plethora of paragraph breaks, images, before & after pictures, and **can be read from front to back in less than an hour.**

However, this book contains **calculations and formulae**, used by most fitness models and bodybuilders, that you will **not** find in most fitness books.

By the time you've finished reading this book, you will know exactly how to achieve that **sexy** body you've been craving for all this time

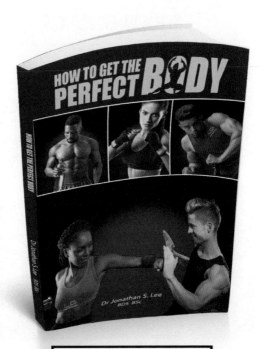

HARDBACK:	N/A
PAPERBACK:	£13.99
E-BOOK:	£9.99

(prices may vary)

AVAILABLE AT
WWW.LEANGAINS.CO.UK
and
Amazon

LEAN MEALS
FOR EVERYONE

Eating regimes and dieting habits vary
massively from one person to the next.
Some dieters, for instance, prefer a
ketogenic approach, whilst others may
prefer to go vegan.

Some trainees prefer a calorie-based
eating regime, whilst others feel more
comfortable fasting for prolonged periods
of time. The point is that one set of fixed
meal plans is very unlikely to cater for
everyone.

Dr Lee wrote **'Lean Meals for Everyone'**
as a means of addressing these issues.

This book contains a wide range of
healthy and nutritious recipes and meal
plans that will suit specific caloric and
nutritional requirements regardless of diet.

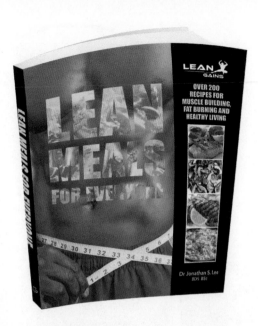

HARDBACK:	N/A
PAPERBACK:	£29.99
E-BOOK:	£9.99

(prices may vary)

AVAILABLE AT
WWW.LEANGAINS.CO.UK
and
Amazon

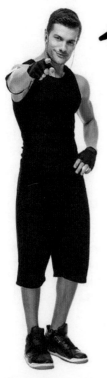

YOUR FEEDBACK IS IMPORTANT TO US!

If you like what you've read, then please take a minute to write a few words on Amazon about this book. I check all my reviews and love to receive feedback.

If you have any queries, questions, or concerns about anything, on the other hand, then please feel free to drop me an email at jon@leangains.co.uk and we will try our best to resolve your issue.

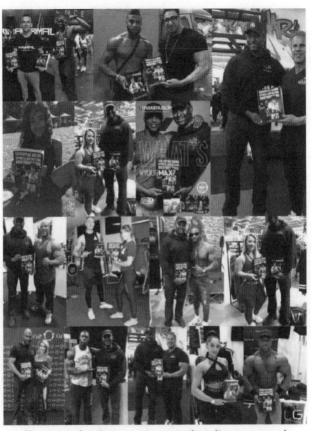

For more books, events, merchandise, personal
trainers, fitness professionals, testimonials,
videos, blogs and upcoming events, then please
visit www.leangains.co.uk

Printed in Great Britain
by Amazon